Top 40 Healthy

Meat Recipes

Learn How to Mix Different Ingredients to Create Tasty Meals

Farrah Richards

Table of Contents

1. Keto Meatloaf

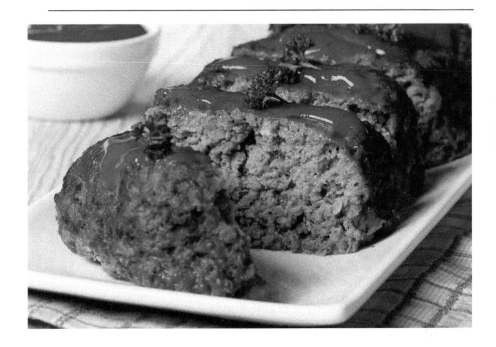

Servings: 8 Slices

Prep Time: 10 Mins

Cook Time: 1 Hr 5 Mins

Total Time: 1 Hr 15 Mins

Ingredients

- 2 pounds 80/20 Ground beef
- 1 medium Onion, diced
- 2 cups Crushed Pork rinds
- 1 large Egg

- 2 tablespoons Worcestershire sauce
- ½ teaspoon Garlic powder
- 1 teaspoon salt
- ⅓ cup Reduced sugar ketchup

Instructions

- Preheat oven to 350 degrees F.
- In a large bowl combine all ingredients except ketchup. Mix ingredients until fully combined.
- Press ingredients into a parchment paper-lined loaf pan.
- Bake for 30 minutes. After 30 minutes add ketchup on top and bake for 25-35 minutes more.
- Remove from oven and let rest for 15 minutes.
- Enjoy!

Nutrition

- Serving: 1slice, Calories: 351kcal, Carbohydrates: 3g, Protein: 25g, Fat: 25g, Saturated Fat: 10g, Cholesterol: 110mg, Sodium: 672mg, Potassium: 369mg, Fiber: 1g, Sugar: 2g, Vitamin A: 34iu, Vitamin C: 2mg, Calcium: 34mg, Iron: 3mg.

2. Quick Chicken Marsala

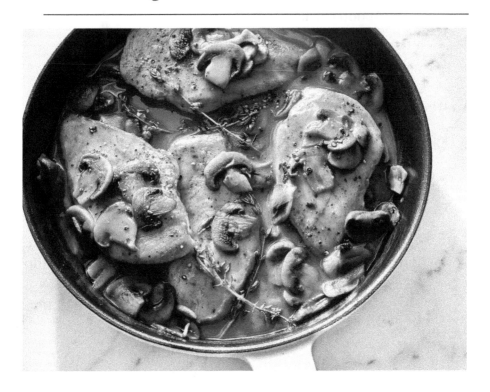

Active Time: 20 Mins

Total Time: 20 Mins

Yield: Serves 4 (serving size: 1 cutlet and about 1/4 cup sauce)

Ingredients

- 2 tablespoons olive oil, divided 4 (4-oz.) skinless, boneless chicken breast cutlets 3/4 teaspoon black pepper, divided 1/2 teaspoon kosher salt, divided 1 (8-oz.) pkg. presliced button mushrooms 4 thyme sprigs 1 tablespoon all-purpose flour 2/3 cup unsalted chicken stock 2/3 cup

Marsala wine 2 1/2 tablespoons unsalted butter 1 tablespoon chopped fresh thyme (optional)

- How To Make It

- Heat 1 tablespoon oil in a large nonstick skillet over medium-high. Sprinkle chicken with 1/2 teaspoon pepper and 1/4 teaspoon salt. Add chicken to pan; cook until done, about 4 minutes per side. Remove chicken from pan (do not wipe out pan).

- Add the remaining 1 tablespoon oil to the pan. Add mushrooms and thyme sprigs; cook, stirring occasionally until mushrooms are browned, about 6 minutes. Sprinkle flour over mixture; cook, stirring constantly, 1 minute.

- Add stock and wine to pan; bring to a boil. Cook until slightly thickened, 2 to 3 minutes. Remove pan from heat. Stir in butter, remaining 1/4 teaspoon pepper, and remaining 1/4 teaspoon salt. Add chicken to pan, turning to coat. Discard thyme sprigs before serving. Sprinkle with chopped thyme, if desired.

Nutrition

- Calories: 344
- Fat:17g
- Satfat: 6g
- Unsat: 9g
- Protein: 28g

- Carbohydrates: 9g
- Fiber: 1g
- Sugars: 7g
- Added sugars: 0g
- Sodium: 567mg
- Calcium: 19g
- Potassium: 16mg

3. Mexican Zucchini And Beef

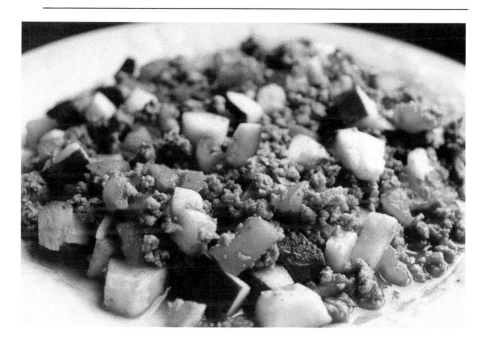

Prep Time: 5 mins

Cook Time: 25 mins

Total Time: 30 mins

Servings: 6 servings

Ingredients

- 2 medium zucchini sliced and quartered
- 1 ½ pounds ground beef
- 2 cloves garlic minced

- 10 ounces mexican style diced tomatoes with green chilis (salsa or diced tomatoes could be used), canned
- 1 tablespoon chili powder
- 1 teaspoon ground cumin
- 1 teaspoon salt
- ½ teaspoon black pepper
- ½ teaspoon onion powder
- ¼ teaspoon crushed red pepper flakes

Instructions

- Brown ground beef with minced garlic, salt, and pepper. Cook over medium heat until meat is browned.
- Add tomatoes and remaining spices. Cover and simmer on low heat for another 10 minutes.
- Add the zucchini. Cover and cook for about 10 more minutes until zucchini is cooked, but still firm.

Nutrition

Serving: 1cup (approx) | Calories: 315 | Carbohydrates: 5g | Protein: 21g | Fat: 23g | Saturated Fat: 9g | Cholesterol: 81mg | Sodium: 498mg | Potassium: 597mg | Fiber: 2g | Sugar: 3g | Vitamin A: 606IU | Vitamin C: 16mg | Calcium: 55mg | Iron: 3mg

4. Low Carb Pho – Vietnamese Beef Noodle Soup

Prep Time: 15 minutes

Cook Time: 3 hours

Total Time: 3 hours 15 minutes

Servings: 5 servings

Ingredients

- The Broth (4-5 servings)
- 5-6 beef soup bones browned and roasted - the more connective tissue, the better!
- 1/2 Onion charred
- 1 tablespoon Fresh Ginger sliced
- 1 tbsp Salt
- 3 tbsp Fish Sauce
- 2 pods Star Anise
- 1 gallon Water

Instructions

- Preheat oven to 425 degrees F.
- Cover beef bones in water and boil for 15 minutes in a large stockpot on the stovetop while the oven preheats. Discard water.

- Place parboiled beef bones and onion on a baking sheet or casserole dish and roast for 45 -60 minutes, until bones are browned and onion is blackened.
- Toss bones, onion, fresh ginger, salt, fish sauce, star anise, and freshwater into the pressure cooker.
- Set pressure cooker to high pressure for 2 hours. If you are using a stovetop, you will simmer for 6-8 hours instead.
- Strain broth with a fine colander.
- Place shirataki noodles and meat of choice in a bowl, pour broth over the top into the bowl while it is still very hot.
- Stir and let sit until raw meat is no longer pink and noodles are cooked 1 to 2 minutes.
- Serve with condiments and veggies of choice on the side.

Nutrition

Calories: 172kcal | Carbohydrates: 3g | Protein: 25g | Fat: 5g | Saturated Fat: 2g | Cholesterol: 67mg | Sodium: 2342mg | Potassium: 461mg | Sugar: 1g | Vitamin A: 135IU | Vitamin C: 5.8mg | Calcium: 62mg | Iron: 2.2mg

5. Instant Pot Low Carb Corned Beef And Cabbage

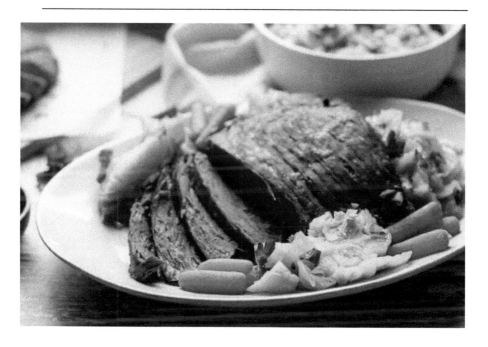

Prep Time: 15 minutes

Cook Time: 1 hour 35 minutes

Total Time: 1 hour 50 minutes

Servings: 8 servings

Ingredients

- 4 pounds corned beef brisket
- 6 cups water
- 2 tsp black peppercorns

- 4 cloves garlic
- 2 tsp dried mustard
- 1 cabbage cut into wedges or 8 cups
- 1 cup onions sliced
- 1 cup carrots sliced into thirds
- 1 cup celery stalks chopped

Instructions

- Place the beef brisket into the pot. Discard the spice packet that comes with the meat.
- Cover the beef with water, add more to cover if needed.
- Add the spices into the pot.
- Cover and set on "Meat/Stew" for 60 minutes on high.
- Hit Cancel then use the Natural Release method, about 20 minutes.
- Remove cover carefully, watch for steam, remove the brisket and keep warm.
- Add the vegetables to the pot and press the "Soup" setting for 15 minutes.
- Use the "Quick" Release method.
- Uncover and add the beef back to the pot to warm through.
- Enjoy immediately!

Nutrition

- Calories: 499

- Calories from Fat: 306
- Fat: 34g
- Saturated Fat: 10g
- Cholesterol: 122mg
- Sodium: 2812mg
- Potassium: 1000mg
- Carbohydrates: 11g
- Fiber: 4g
- Sugar: 5g
- Protein: 35g
- Vitamin A: 2840IU
- Vitamin C: 106.1mg
- Calcium: 89mg
- Iron: 4.6mg

6. Korean Ground Beef Recipe

Prep Time: 10 mins

Cook Time: 10 mins

Total Time: 20 mins

Ingredients

Sauce:

- ¼ cup reduced-sodium soy sauce (or use a gluten-free alternative and add salt as needed)
- 1 tablespoon honey or a liquid sugar-free alternative
- 1 teaspoon cornstarch
- ½ teaspoon crushed red pepper flakes

Stir-Fry:

- 2 tablespoons avocado oil
- 1 lb. lean ground beef (85/15)
- 1 tablespoon minced fresh garlic
- 1 tablespoon minced fresh ginger root

To Finish The Dish:

- 1 tablespoon sesame oil
- ¼ cup thinly sliced green onions, green parts only

Instructions

- In a small bowl, prepare the sauce by whisking together the soy sauce, honey, cornstarch, and red pepper flakes. Set aside. In a large skillet, heat the oil over medium-high heat.
- Add the beef and cook, stirring, until no longer pink, breaking it up into crumbles as you cook, about 5 minutes.
- Drain the beef. Return to the skillet. Add the garlic and the ginger to the skillet and cook, stirring, for 1 minute.
- Stir the sauce into the beef. Cook 2 more minutes, until heated through and the sauce thickens.
- Off heat, drizzle the dish with sesame oil, sprinkle it with green onions, and serve.

Nutrition

- Calories: 370
- Fat: 27g
- Saturated Fat: 8g
- Sodium: 651mg
- Carbohydrates: 7g
- Fiber: 0.3g
- Sugar: 4g
- Protein: 22g

7. Beef Tenderloin

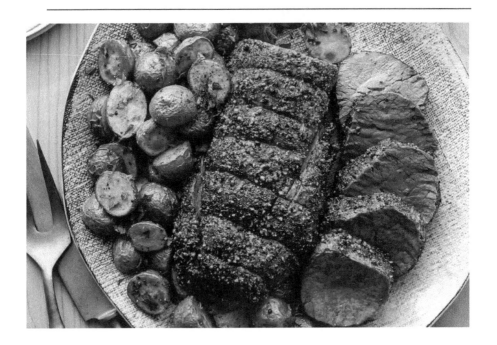

Prep Time: 15 mins

Cook Time: 45 mins

Total Time: 1 hr

Ingredients

- 1 beef tenderloin Plan two 2″ filets per person
- 1 tablespoon Stone House Seasoning Recipe

Instructions

- Place beef tenderloin on a rimmed baking sheet, pat dry with paper towels, and season both sides of the meat with

Stone House Seasoning. Cover tightly with plastic wrap and refrigerate for one hour or up to 4 days before you plan on cooking and serving.

- Remove from the refrigerator, unwrap and allow to stand for about an hour to come to room temperature.
- Meanwhile, preheat grill or oven to approximately 400° F.
- Place tenderloin onto the grill or in the oven. Allow the beef tenderloin to cook until it reaches 145° F when checked with an internal meat thermometer in the thinner areas and 140° F in the thicker area, about 45 minutes.
- Remove from grill and cover loosely with aluminum foil and allow to rest on the carving board for about 15 minutes before carving and serving.

Nutrition

Calories: 238kcal | Protein: 35g | Fat: 10g | Saturated Fat: 1g | Cholesterol: 105mg | Sodium: 64mg

8. Simple Beef Stroganoff

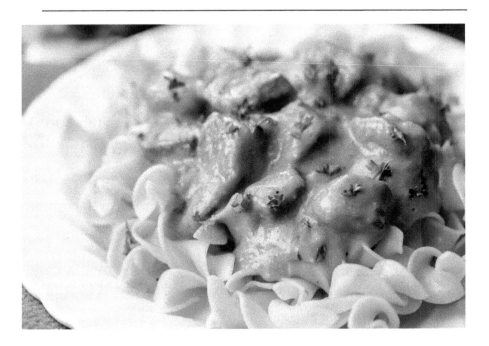

Prep Time: 5 mins

Cook Time: 25 mins

Total Time: 30 mins

Servings: 6

Ingredients

- 1 tablespoon olive oil
- 2 pounds beef (roast, sirloin, or beef tenderloin) sliced into 1/4-inch slices
- 1 teaspoon Stone House Seasoning

- 1 cup sour cream
- 1 package egg noodles cooked according to package directions

Instructions

- Add olive oil to a medium skillet (or Dutch oven) set over medium heat. Add beef slices and sprinkle with Stone House Seasoning. Cook the beef until browned and cooked for about 8 minutes.
- Stir in the sour cream until smooth to make the sauce.
- Serve over egg noodles or mashed potatoes. You can also add the egg noodles to the skillet or Dutch oven and mix them into the sauce if you prefer. Top with fresh parsley, if using.

Nutrition

Calories: 584kcal | Carbohydrates: 41g | Protein: 38g | Fat: 30g | Saturated Fat: 13g | Cholesterol: 172mg | Sodium: 553mg | Potassium: 694mg | Fiber: 2g | Sugar: 2g | Vitamin A: 294IU | Vitamin C: 1mg | Calcium: 88mg | Iron: 4mg

9. Perfect Prime Rib Recipe

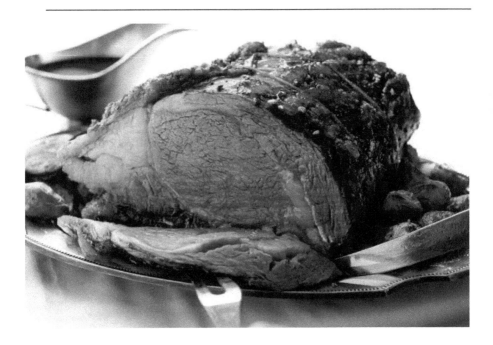

Prep Time: 1 hr

Cook Time: 2 hrs

Resting Time: 20 mins

Total Time: 3 hrs

Ingredients

- 1 (3 – 4 bone) bone-in prime rib, about (10 – 10.5 pounds)
- 1 tablespoon kosher salt
- 2 teaspoons freshly ground black pepper

Instructions

- Salt prime rib from one hour to up to five days before cooking and serving your prime rib. Once salted, wrap tightly in plastic wrap and refrigerate until an hour before cooking.

- An hour before cooking, remove the prime rib from the refrigerator, unwrap and place, bone side down, on a roasting pan and allow to reach room temperature. If cooking a boneless roast, place onto a roasting rack inside the roasting pan. At this point add pepper or other seasonings, if using.

- Preheat oven to 475° F. Then, roast your prime rib for 15 minutes and reduce to 325° F until your prime rib reaches the desired internal temperature, usually 11 – 12 minutes per pound, about 1 hour and 50 minutes. Using an internal meat thermometer, remove your prime rib from the oven about 2 – 4 degrees less than the desired serving final temperature you desire. The temperature of the prime rib will continue to rise due to carryover cooking. Tent prime rib with foil and allow to rest for 20 minutes.

- Place on a carving board for slicing and serve.

Nutrition

Serving: 3ounces | Calories: 340kcal | Protein: 19g | Fat: 29g | Saturated Fat: 12g | Polyunsaturated Fat: 1g | Monounsaturated Fat: 12g | Cholesterol: 72mg | Sodium: 55mg | Potassium: 258mg

10.   Cola Glazed Ham Recipe

Prep Time: 5 mins

Cook Time: 1 hr

Total Time: 1 hr 5 mins

Servings: 16

Ingredients

- 1 (8-pound) fully cooked, spiral-sliced ham
- 1 (12-ounce) can Coca-Cola
- 1 cup brown sugar firmly packed

Instructions

- Preheat oven to 325° F. Place ham in a roasting pan. Combine Coca-Cola and brown sugar and pour over ham. Cover tightly with aluminum foil. Every 30 minutes, uncover the ham and baste well with the pan juices and then recover the ham. Bake 20 minutes per pound, until the thickest part of the ham registers 140° F on a meat thermometer, about 2 hours. Remove the foil for the last 10 minutes of cooking time so that after the final glaze, the glaze can caramelize on the ham
- Remove roasting pan from the oven and baste again. Let the ham stand for about 15 minutes, remove the ham from the roasting pan and onto a platter for serving.

Nutrition

Calories: 52kcal | Carbohydrates: 13g | Sodium: 4mg | Potassium: 18mg | Sugar: 13g | Calcium: 11mg | Iron: 0.1mg

11. Hamburger Sliders With A Spicy Cilantro Lime Spread

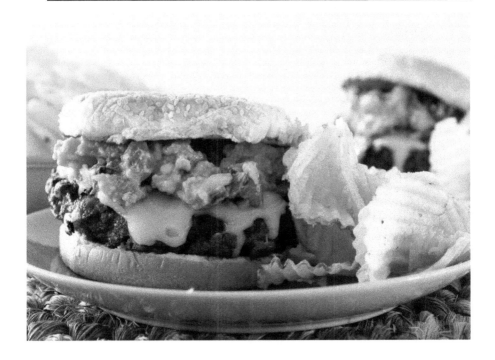

Prep Time: 10 mins

Cook Time: 15 mins

Total Time: 25 mins

Ingredients

- 1 pound ground beef
- 1 clove garlic minced
- 1 tablespoon worcestershire sauce
- 1/2 cup mayonnaise

- 1/4 cup cilantro
- 2 tablespoons lime juice
- 4 dashes of tabasco sauce
- Salt and pepper
- Slider buns or rolls
- Lettuce
- Cheese
- Tomato

Instructions

- Mix ground beef, garlic, and Worcestershire sauce until well-combined.
- Form into 8 small patties. Refrigerate until ready to cook.
- Blend mayonnaise, cilantro, lime juice, Tabasco sauce, salt, and pepper until creamy. Adjust to your taste preference.
- Cook hamburger patties. Open slider buns or rolls and spread spicy cilantro-lime spread on top and bottom of the bun.
- Add hamburger patty and lettuce, cheese, and tomato.
- Serve warm.

Nutrition

Calories: 484kcal | Carbohydrates: 1g | Protein: 19g | Fat: 43g | Saturated Fat: 11g | Cholesterol: 92mg | Sodium:

296mg | Potassium: 340mg | Sugar: 1g | Vitamin A: 85IU | Vitamin C: 3.3mg | Calcium: 25mg | Iron: 2.5mg

12.   Skillet Pork Chop Recipe

Prep Time: 5 mins

Cook Time: 25 mins

Total Time: 30 mins

Ingredients

- 6-8 Pork Chops Bone-In, Thick Sliced
- 2-3 Tablespoons Olive Oil
- Salt
- Pepper

Instructions

- preheat oven to 350 degrees.
- Pour olive oil into a skillet over medium heat.
- Add pork chops and season with salt and pepper.
- Cook about 3-5 minutes on each side, until each side has browned well.
- Place skillet in the oven for about 15 minutes.
- Serve immediately.

Nutrition

Calories: 249kcal | Protein: 29g | Fat: 14g | Saturated Fat: 4g | Cholesterol: 90mg | Sodium: 64mg | Potassium: 500mg | Calcium: 9mg | Iron: 1mg

13.   One Pot Penne Pasta Recipe

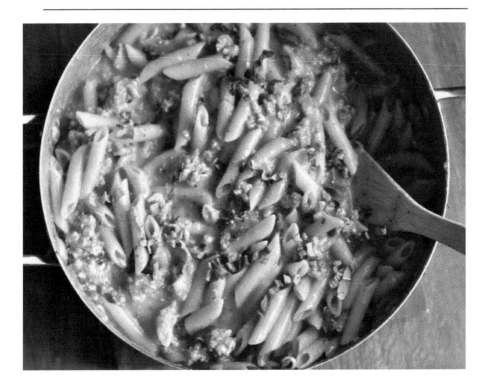

Prep Time: 5 mins

Cook Time: 10 mins

Total Time: 15 mins

Ingredients

- 1 pound smoked sausage cut into bite-sized slices
- 1/2 medium onion diced
- 2 cloves garlic minced
- 1 cup sliced mushrooms

- 3 cups penne pasta uncooked
- 2 cups chicken stock or broth
- 1 (10-ounce) jar roasted red peppers undrained
- 2 cups Monterey Jack cheese
- 1/2 cup Parmesan cheese
- 2 cups fresh spinach

Instructions

- Add sausage, onions, garlic, and mushrooms to a medium pot over medium heat. Cook until onions are slightly tender, stirring often. Add in penne pasta, chicken stock, roasted red peppers, along with the liquid from the jar. Stir to combine and cover for about 5-8 minutes. Remove lid, stir and continue to cook until penne pasta is al dente or at the amount of tenderness you prefer.
- Stir in the cheeses and fresh spinach until well combined and the spinach is tender. Serve.

Nutrition

Calories: 482kcal | Carbohydrates: 36g | Protein: 23g | Fat: 26g | Saturated Fat: 11g | Cholesterol: 71mg | Sodium: 822mg | Potassium: 302mg | Fiber: 1g | Sugar: 2g | Vitamin A: 265IU | Vitamin C: 0.8mg | Calcium: 302mg | Iron: 1.5mg

14. Chili Rubbed Chicken Skewers Recipe

Prep Time: 10 mins

Cook Time: 10 mins

Total Time: 20 mins

Servings: 4 servings

Ingredients

- 2 chicken breasts boneless, skinless, and cut into 1-inch pieces
- 1 teaspoon Stone House Seasoning
- 1 teaspoon chili powder
- 1/2 teaspoon paprika
- 1/2 teaspoon cumin
- pinch cayenne pepper
- 2 medium red peppers cut into 1-inch pieces
- 1 small red onion cut into 1-inch pieces
- 4 medium zucchini cut into 1-inch pieces

Instructions

- Place the chicken pieces into a large zip-top bag. Add Stone House Seasoning, chili powder, paprika, cumin, and cayenne pepper to the chicken. Remove as much air as possible as you are sealing the bag. Massage the seasoning onto the chicken, making sure that each piece is coated. Place into the refrigerator until ready to build your skewers.

- Build your skewers by alternating vegetable pieces with the chili-rubbed chicken. (Zucchini, chicken, pepper, chicken, onion, chicken, and zucchini works well as the zucchini holds the skewer ingredients in place.)
- Preheat the grill, grill pan, or skillet to medium heat. Spray or brush with olive oil spray.
- Cook the chili-rubbed chicken skewers on the grill, grill pan, or skillet for five minutes. Flip and cook an additional five minutes or until the chicken has cooked through.

Nutrition

Calories: 183kcal | Carbohydrates: 10g | Protein: 27g | Fat: 3g | Cholesterol: 72mg | Sodium: 157mg | Potassium: 1064mg | Fiber: 3g | Sugar: 7g | Vitamin A: 2560IU | Vitamin C: 112.4mg | Calcium: 41mg | Iron: 1.7mg

15. Slow Cooker Beef Bourguignon Recipe

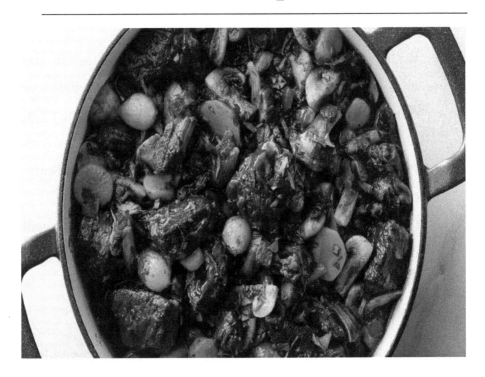

Prep Time:10 mins

Cook Time: 6 hrs

Total Time: 6 hrs 10 mins

Servings: 6

Ingredients

- 3 slices bacon diced
- 1 3-4 pound chuck roast, cut into 2-inch cubes

- 1 1/2 tablespoons all-purpose flour
- 1 1/2 teaspoons stone house seasoning plus more to taste
- 2 cups sliced mushrooms
- 2 cups about 3 medium sliced carrots
- 2 cups about 3 medium diced red potatoes
- 1 medium onion peeled and cut into 2-inch chunks
- 2 tablespoons tomato paste
- 4 stalks fresh thyme
- 2 bay leaves
- 1 cup red wine
- 4 cups beef stock or broth
- Fresh parsley optional garnish

Instructions

- Cook bacon until crispy in stove top-compatible slow cooker insert or a skillet set over medium heat. Using a slotted spoon, remove the bacon from the slow cooker insert (or skillet) and set it aside. Add the beef to the bacon drippings, along with the flour and Stone House Seasoning. Stir to coat the beef and then cook the beef until it is well-browned about 6 minutes.
- Transfer the slow cooker insert over to the slow cooker and add bacon to your bacon. If you do not have a stove top-compatible insert, you'll transfer the crispy bacon and cooked beef from your skillet into the slow cooker.

- Add in the mushrooms, carrots, onions, red potatoes, and onion. Then, add the tomato paste, fresh thyme, bay leaves, burgundy (or your favorite hearty red wine), and beef broth. Set timer for 6 to 8 hours on the low setting.

Nutrition

Serving: 2cups | Calories: 506kcal | Carbohydrates: 13.9g | Protein: 63.2g | Fat: 17.6g | Saturated Fat: 5.4g | Fiber: 2g | Sugar: 3.6g

16.   Balsamic Roast Beef Recipe

Prep Time: 5 mins

Cook Time: 4 hrs

Total Time: 4 hrs 5 mins

Ingredients

- 1 (3-4 pound) boneless roast beef (chuck or round roast)
- 1 cup beef stock or broth
- 1/2 cup balsamic vinegar
- 1 tablespoon Worcestershire sauce
- 1 tablespoon soy sauce
- 1 tablespoon honey
- 1/2 teaspoon red pepper flakes
- 4 cloves garlic chopped

Instructions

- Place roast beef into the insert of your slow cooker. In a 2-cup measuring cup, mix all remaining ingredients. Pour over roast beef and set the timer for your slow cooker. (4 hours on High or 6-8 hours on Low)
- Once roast beef has cooked, remove it from the slow cooker with tongs into a serving dish. Break apart lightly with two forks and then ladle about 1/4 - 1/2 cup of gravy over roast beef.

- Store remaining gravy in an airtight container in the refrigerator for another use.

Nutrition

Calories: 432kcal | Carbohydrates: 6g | Protein: 43g | Fat: 35g | Saturated Fat: 1g | Cholesterol: 1mg | Sodium: 181mg | Potassium: 57mg | Fiber: 1g | Sugar: 5g | Vitamin A: 37IU | Vitamin C: 1mg | Calcium: 11mg | Iron: 1mg

17.   Garlic Roasted Pork Chops

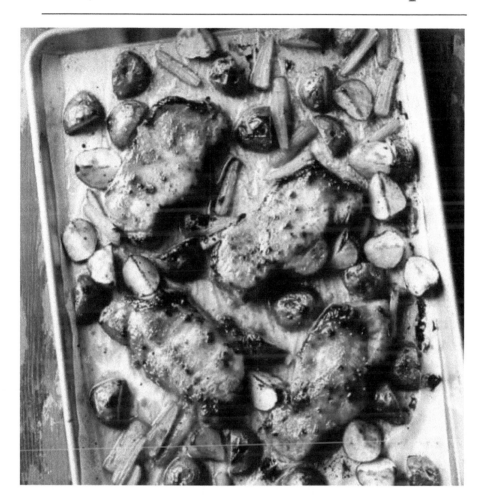

Prep Time: 10 mins

Cook Time: 15 mins

Total Time: 25 mins

Ingredients

- 1 tbsp olive oil
- 1 tsp sea salt
- 1/2 tsp ground black pepper
- 4 boneless center-cut pork chops
- 6-8 cloves garlic, peeled and whole

Instructions

- Heat the oven to 400 degrees.
- In an oven-safe skillet, heat the olive oil over high heat.
- Season the pork chops with salt and pepper.
- Once the oil is hot, add the pork chops to the skillet and sear for 2-3 minutes, until golden brown.
- Flip the chops over, toss in the garlic cloves, and place the pan in the hot oven.
- Roast the chops for 2 minutes.
- Then, carefully flip the chops and the garlic over and roast for another 2 minutes, or until they are cooked through.
- Carefully remove from the oven. Allow the chops to rest, out of the hot pan, for about 5 minutes, and then serve. Serve the roasted garlic alongside.

Nutrition

Fat:4.5g|SaturatedFat:1g|Cholesterol:5.1mg|Sodium:693.6mg|Carbohydrates 31.9g|Fiber 0.2g|Sugar 0.1g|Protein 39g

18.   Mediterranean Pork Loin With Sun-Dried Tomatoes And Olives

Prep Time: 5 Minutes

Cook Time: 240 Minutes

Total Time: 245 Minutes

Servings: 4-6 Serving

Ingredients

- 11/2-2 lbs pork tenderloin (NOT marinated)
- 1 C Broth of your choice (chicken, vegetable, etc.)
- 2 teaspoons Garlic, chives, lemon, salt, pepper, onion, and garlic powder)
- 1/2 teaspoon s Mediterranean Seasoning
- 10 green olives, sliced
- 1 T sun-dried tomatoes (not in oil) sliced thin

Instructions

- Place pork loin in the bottom of the Crock-Pot (slow cooker.)
- Pour the broth over the meat.
- Sprinkle with the seasonings, then scatter the olives and sun-dried tomatoes around the meat.

- Place the lid on and cook on high for 4 hours, or low for 6 hours. Meat may need longer if frozen. It will be done when the internal temperature reaches 155 degrees F.
- Slice the meat thin, drizzle with some of the broth, and garnish with a few olive and sun-dried tomato pieces.
- Serve hot.

Nutrition

- Calories: 210
- Total Fat: 5.6g
- Sat Fat: 1.8g
- Cholesterol: 103mg
- Sodium: 155mg
- Carbohydrates: 0.7g
- Fiber: 0.2g
- Sugar: 0g
- Protein: 37.2g
- Calcium: 18mg
- Iron:2mg
- Potassium: 600mg

19.   Tex Mex Turkey Stuffed Poblanos

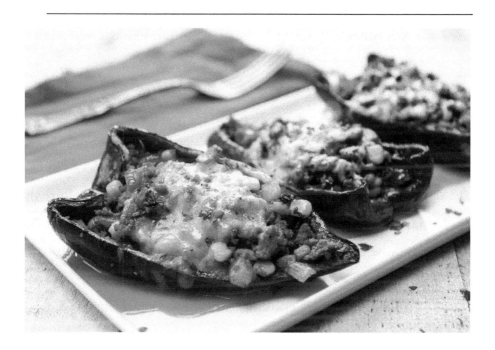

Prep Time: 15 Minutes

Cook Time: 20 Minutes

Total Time: 35 Minutes

Servings: 4 Serving

Ingredients

- 2 large poblano peppers (or bell peppers) cut in half lengthwise and seeds removed
- 4 tsp (or fresh garlic and oil of your choice)

- 2 pounds ground turkey, 98% lean
- 1 T (one capful) or Phoenix Sunrise Seasoning (or garlic, onion, cilantro, cumin, and black pepper)
- 1 C reduced-fat extra sharp cheddar cheese, shredded (divided)
- 8 T sour cream
- Fresh cilantro and/or sliced jalapenos for garnish

Instructions

- Preheat the oven to 350 degrees. Spray a casserole dish large enough to hold the pepper halves with nonstick cooking spray and place the peppers, cut side up into the dish. Bake for 15 minutes.
- While peppers are cooking, add the Roasted Garlic Oil to a large skillet and heat over medium-high heat.
- Add turkey to the pan and sprinkle with the seasoning. Cook for 10 minutes, stirring occasionally until turkey is browned.
- Remove meat from the heat and stir in 1/2 C of the cheddar cheese.
- Remove the peppers from the oven and place equal portions of the meat into the pepper halves. Sprinkle with remaining cheese and bake until poblanos are tender and cheese is melted for about 5-7 additional minutes.
- Drizzle 2 T of sour cream over each pepper and sprinkle with cilantro and/or jalapenos if desired.

Nutrition

- Calories: 357
- Total Fat: 14.4g
- Sat Fat: 7.3g
- Cholesterol: 140mg
- Sodium: 324mg
- Carbohydrates: 4.1g
- Fiber: 0.3g
- Sugar: 1.2g
- Protein: 55g
- Calcium: 397mg
- Iron: 2mg
- Potassium: 705mg

20.   Classic Beef Barley Soup

Prep Time: 15 Minutes

Cook Time: 45 Minutes

Total Time: 1 Hour

Servings: 8 Servings

Ingredients

- 1 tablespoon olive oil
- 2 1/2 - 3 pounds beef chuck roast
- 1 large sweet onion, peeled and chopped
- 2 cups sliced carrots
- 2 cups sliced celery
- 4 cloves garlic, minced
- 12 cups beef broth
- 15 ounces fire-roasted diced tomatoes (1 can)
- 1 cup dried barley
- 1 tablespoon fresh thyme leaves (1 teaspoon dried)
- 1 tablespoon freshly chopped rosemary leaves (1 teaspoon dried)
- 1/2 teaspoon crushed red pepper
- Salt and pepper

Instructions

- Place a large saucepot over medium heat and add the olive oil and onions. Saute the onions for 2-3 minutes. Then stir in the carrots, celery, and garlic. Cook for another 3-5 minutes.
- Meanwhile, cut the beef into small 1/2-inch chunks. Push the veggies to the side of the pot and add the meat. Brown for 5 minutes, stirring once or twice. Then add in the broth, tomatoes, barley, herbs, crushed red pepper, and 1/2 teaspoon salt. Stir well.
- Cover the pot and bring to a boil. Lower the heat if needed and simmer until the barley is cooked and the beef is tender, stirring occasionally. About 30 minutes.
- Taste. Then season with salt and pepper as needed.

Nutrition

Calories: 373kcal, Carbohydrates: 27g, Protein: 30g, Fat: 16g, Saturated Fat: 6g, Cholesterol: 78mg, Sodium: 1563mg, Potassium: 903mg, Fiber: 6g, Sugar: 5g, Vitamin C: 7.7mg, Calcium: 103mg, Iron: 4.6mg

21.   Low-Carb Beef Stroganoff

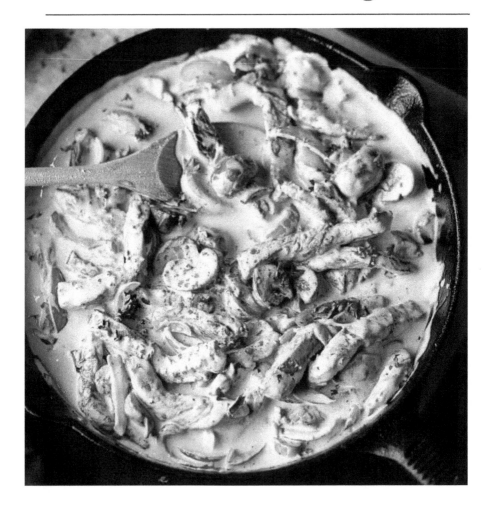

Servings: 4

Ingredients:

- 1 1/2 lb beef tenderloin -- thin strips
- 2 tbsp all-purpose flour
- 2 tbsp butter
- 2 tbsp olive oil

- 1 1/2 cups beef bouillon
- 1/4 cup sour cream
- 2 tbsp tomato paste
- 1/2 tsp paprika
- salt to taste

Directions

1. Dredge beef in flour.
2. In a heavy skillet, melt butter with oil.
3. Brown the beef (about 5 minutes).
4. Slowly add bouillon to beef, stirring well.
5. Bring to a boil.
6. Combine sour cream, tomato paste, paprika, and salt. Slowly stir sour cream mixture into beef mixture.
7. Turn heat to low and bring to a bare simmer. Cook 15-20 minutes, stirring frequently and never allowing mixture to boil.

22.   Indian Red Curry

Servings: 4

Ingredients:

- 1 lb beef stew
- 1 tbsp butter
- 1/2 tsp curry paste -- or powder
- 1 dash cinnamon,cardamom, and pepper
- 1 cup canned coconut milk
- 1/2 cup red pepper
- 1 tsp paprika
- 1 garlic clove

Directions

1. Brown meat and garlic in butter, then add spices and stir fry few minutes.
2. Add red pepper and coconut milk.
3. Reduce heat and simmer til done (2-3 hours, add water if necessary.)

23.   Corned Beef and Cabbage

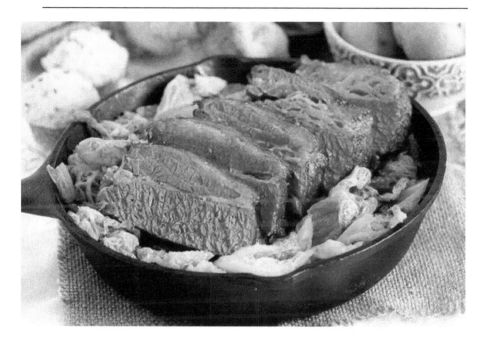

Servings: 6

Ingredients:

- 4 cups Hot Water
- 2 tbsp Cider Vinegar
- 2 tbsp Splenda
- 1/2 tsp Pepper -- Freshly Ground
- 1 Large Onion -- Cut Into Wedges
- 3 lb Corned Beef -- 1.5kg With Spices
- 1 Cabbage
- Cored And Cut into 10 Wedges

Directions

1. In a 6 quart – 6 litre crock pot, combine the water, vinegar, splenda, pepper, and onions, mixing well.
2. Place the corned beef into the mixture.
3. Cover and cook on high heat for 4 hours.
4. Remove the lid and scatter the cabbage wedges over the top.
5. Cover and continue cooking on high 3 to 4 hours longer, or until the beef is tender.
6. To serve, carve the beef into slices and serve with the cabbage, with some of the cooking liquid spooned over the beef to keep it moist.

Nutritional Facts

248 Calories 20g Fat (70.5% calories from fat)

9g Protein 10g Carbohydrate 2g Dietary Fiber

35mg Cholesterol 522mg Sodium

24.   Barbecue Meat Loaf

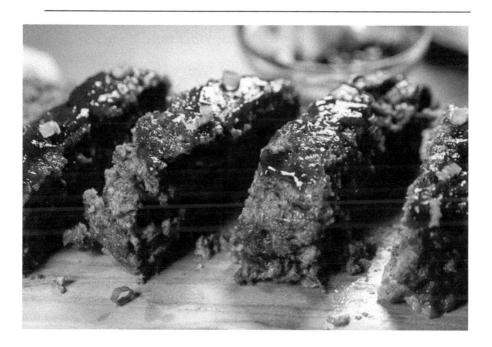

Yield: 6 servings

Ingredients:

- 1/4 cup (40 g) onion, finely chopped
- 1/4 cup (25 g) celery, finely chopped
- 1/4 cup (60 g) low-sodium catsup
- 1 egg
- 1/4 cup (30 g) dry bread crumbs
- 1 teaspoon (5 ml) liquid smoke
- Dash black pepper
- 11/2 pounds (680 g) lean ground beef

Directions:

1. Place all ingredients except beef in mixing bowl and mix well.
2. Add beef to catsup mixture and mix until blended.
3. Shape into a loaf about 3112 x 7-inch (9 x 18 cm).
4. Place in a pan that has been sprayed with nonstick vegetable oil spray or lined with aluminum foil.
5. Bake at 325°F (170°C, or gas mark 3) about 1 hour or until browned and firm.
6. Pour off any fat and drippings and let set for 10 minutes before cutting into 6 equal slices.

Nutritional Info:94 g water; 311 calories (61 % from fat, 30% from protein, 9% from carb); 23 g Protein; 21 g total fat; 8 g

25. Home-Style Meat Loaf

Yield: 6 servings

Ingredients:

- 3/4 cup (180 g) ketchup, divided
- 1/2 cup (40 g) quick-cooking oats
- 1/4 cup (40 g) minced onion
- 2 tablespoons (8 g) chopped parsley
- 1 tablespoon (1 5 g) brown sugar
- 1/4 teaspoon black pepper
- 2 large egg whites, lightly beaten
- 11/2 pounds (680 g) ground round

Directions:

1. Preheat oven to 350°F (180°C, gas mark 4).
2. Combine 112 cup (120 g) ketchup, oats, and next 6 ingredients (oats through egg whites) in a large bowl.
3. Add meat; stir just until blended.
4. Shape meat mixture into an 8 x 4-inch (20 x 10 cm) loaf on a broiler pan coated with nonstick vegetable oil spray.
5. Brush remaining ketchup over meat loaf. Bake 11/2 hours or until done.

Nutritional Info:110 g water; 363 calories (51 % from fat, 28% from protein, 21 % from carb); 25 g protein; 20 g total fat; 8 g

26.   German Meatballs

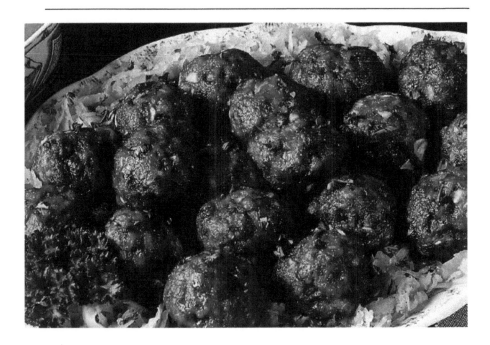

Yield: 6 servings

Ingredients:

- 1 egg
- 1/4 cup (60 ml) skim milk
- 1/4 cup (30 g) bread crumbs
- 1/4 teaspoon poultry seasoning
- 1 pound (455 g) extra-lean ground beef
- 2 cups (475 ml) low-sodium beef broth
- 1/2 cup (35 g) sliced mushrooms
- 1/2 cup (80 g) chopped onion
- 1 cup (230 g) fat-free sour cream

- 1 tablespoon (8 g) flour
- 1 teaspoon caraway seed

Directions:

1. Combine egg and milk.
2. Stir in crumbs and seasoning.
3. Add meat and mix well.
4. Form into 24 meatballs, about 11/2 inches (31/2 cm).
5. Brown meatballs in skillet.
6. Drain. Add broth, mushrooms, and onion. Cover and simmer for 30 minutes.
7. Stir together sour cream, flour, and caraway seed. Stir into skillet.
8. Cook and stir until thickened.

Nutritional Info:194 g water; 281 calories (32% from fat, 47% from protein, 21 % from carb); 19 g protein; 6 g total fat; 2 g

27.   Zucchini Stuffed Pork Chops

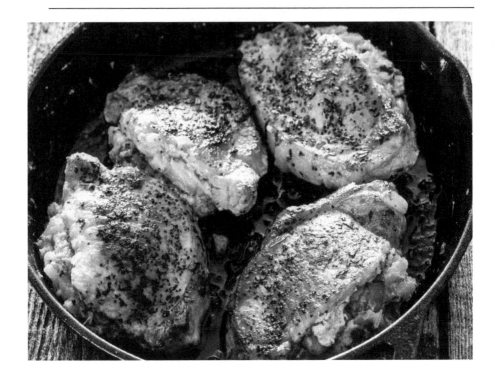

Yeld: 4 Serving

Ingredients:

- 11/2 cup (188 g) zucchini, shredded
- 1 clove garlic, crushed
- 2 tablespoons (10 g) parmesan cheese, grated
- 1/4 teaspoon black pepper
- 4 boneless pork loin chops
- 1 teaspoon (5 ml) olive oil
- 1/2 cup (120 ml) dry white wine or chicken broth

- 1 tablespoon (11 g) Dijon mustard

Directions:

1. Squeeze zucchini with paper towels to remove moisture.
2. Spray 10-inch (25 cm) nonstick skillet with nonstick cooking spray.
3. Cook zucchini and garlic in skillet over medium heat about 3 minutes or until tender. Stir in cheese and pepper.
4. Remove zucchini mixture from skillet; cool.
5. Trim fat from pork chops.
6. Flatten each pork chop to 1/4-inch (5 mm) thickness between waxed paper or plastic wrap.
7. Spread one-fourth of the zucchini mixture over each piece of pork.
8. Roll up; secure with wooden picks.
9. Add oil and pork rolls to skillet. Cover and cook over medium heat 15 to 20 minutes, turning once, until done.
10. Remove wooden picks. Remove pork rolls from skillet; keep warm.
11. Add wine to skillet.
12. Cook over high heat 2 to 3 minutes or until reduced by half. Stir in mustard. Pour sauce over pork rolls.

Nutritional Info: 148 g water; 187 calories (36% from fat, 57% from protein, 7% from carb); 23 g Protein; 7 9 total fat; 2 g

28.   Pork Chops in Onion Sauce

Yeld: 4 Serving

Ingredients:

- 4 pork loin chops
- 1/4 teaspoon pepper
- 11/2 tablespoons (12 g) flour
- 11/2 tablespoons (25 ml) olive oil
- 4 small onions, thinly sliced
- 1/2 cup (120 ml) beer
- 1/2 cup (120 ml) low-sodium beef broth
- 1 teaspoon cornstarch

Directions:

1. Season pork chops with pepper; coat with flour.
2. Heat oil in a heavy skillet.
3. Add pork chops; fry for 3 minutes on each side. Add onions; cook for another 5 minutes, turning chops once.
4. Pour in beer and beef broth; cover and simmer 15 minutes.
5. Remove pork shops to a preheated platter.
6. Blend cornstarch with a small amount of cold water.
7. Stir into sauce and cook until thick and bubbly.
8. Pour over pork chops.

Nutritional Info: 238 g water; 250 calories (36% from fat, 39% from protein, 25% from carb); 23 g Protein; 10 g total fat; 2 g

29.   Ham and Artichoke Hearts Scalloped Potatoes

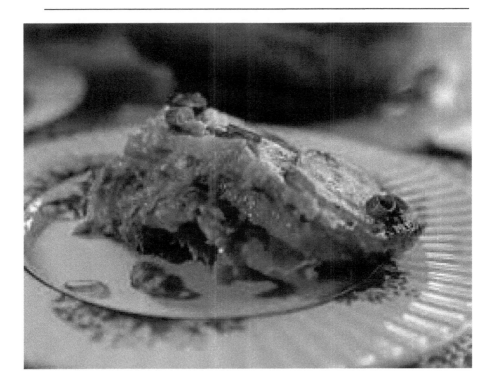

Serves 4

Ingredients:

- 2 cups frozen artichoke hearts
- Nonstick spray
- 1 cup chopped onion
- 4 small potatoes, thinly sliced
- Sea salt and freshly ground black pepper to taste (optional)

- 1 tablespoon lemon juice
- 1 tablespoon dry white wine
- 1 cup Mock Cream (see recipe in Chapter 6)
- ½ cup nonfat cottage cheese
- 1 teaspoon dried parsley
- 1 teaspoon garlic powder
- ½cup freshly grated Parmesan cheese
- ½ pound (4 ounces) cubed lean ham
- 2 ounces grated Cheddar cheese (to yield ½ cup)

Directions:

1. Preheat oven to 300°F.

2. Thaw artichoke hearts and pat dry with a paper towel. In deep casserole dish treated with nonstick spray, layer artichokes, onion, and potatoes; lightly sprinkle salt and pepper over top (if using).

3. In a food processor or blender, combine lemon juice, wine, Mock Cream, cottage cheese, parsley, garlic powder, and Parmesan cheese; process until smooth. Pour over

layered vegetables; top with ham. Cover casserole dish (with a lid or foil); bake 35– 40 minutes or until potatoes are cooked through.

1. Remove cover; top with Cheddar cheese. Return to oven another 10 minutes or until cheese is melted and bubbly. Let rest 10 minutes before cutting.

Nutritional Analysis (per serving, without salt):

Calories: 269 Protein: 21g Carbohydrates: 31g Fat: 8g Saturated Fat: 4g Cholesterol: 28mg Sodium: 762mg Fiber: 6g

30.　Italian Sausage

Yields about 2 pounds

Ingredients:

- 2 pounds (32 ounces) pork shoulder
- 1 teaspoon ground black pepper
- 1 teaspoon dried parsley
- 1 teaspoon Italian-style seasoning
- 1 teaspoon garlic powder
- 3/4 teaspoon crushed anise seeds
- 1/8 teaspoon red pepper flakes
- ½ teaspoon paprika
- ½ teaspoon instant minced onion flakes
- 1 teaspoon kosher or sea salt (optional)

Directions:

1. Remove all fat from meat; cut the meat into cubes. Put in food processor; grind to desired consistency.

2. Add remaining ingredients; mix until well blended. You can put sausage mixture in casings, but it works equally well broiled or grilled as patties.

Nutritional Analysis (per serving, without salt):

Calories: 135 Protein: 15g Carbohydrates: 0g Fat: 8g Saturated Fat: 3g Cholesterol: 45mg Sodium: 27mg Fiber: 0g

31.   Italian Sweet Fennel Sausage

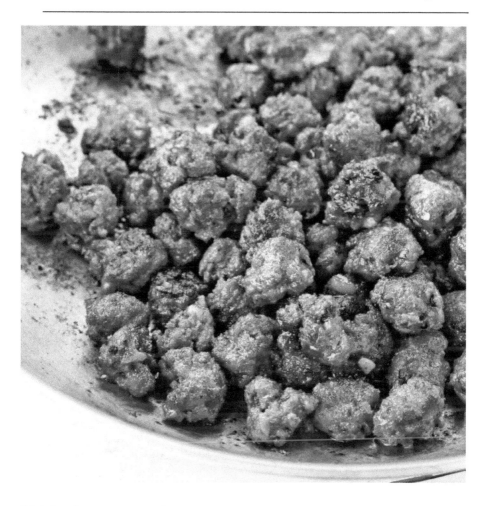

Yields about 2 pounds

Ingredients:

- 1 tablespoon fennel seeds
- ¼ teaspoon ground cayenne pepper
- 2 pounds (32 ounces) pork butt

- ½ teaspoon black pepper
- 2 ½ teaspoons crushed garlic
- 1 tablespoon sugar

Directions:

1. Toast fennel seeds and cayenne pepper in nonstick skillet over medium heat, stirring constantly, until seeds just begin to darken, about 2 minutes. Set aside.

2. Remove all fat from meat; cut the meat into cubes. Put in food processor; grind to desired consistency.

3. Add fennel and cayenne mixture plus remaining ingredients; mix until well blended.

4. You can put sausage mixture in casings, but it works equally well broiled or grilled as patties.

Nutritional Analysis (per serving, without salt):

Calories: 139 Protein: 15g Carbohydrates: 1g Fat: 8g Saturated Fat: 3g Cholesterol: 45mg Sodium: 27mg Fiber: 0g

32.   Mock Chorizo

Yields about 2 pounds

Ingredients:

- 2 pounds (32 ounces) lean pork
- 4 tablespoons chili powder
- ¼ teaspoon ground cloves
- 2 tablespoons paprika
- 2 ½ teaspoons crushed fresh garlic
- 1 teaspoon crushed dried oregano
- 3 ½ tablespoons cider vinegar
- 1 teaspoon kosher or sea salt (optional)

Directions:

1. Remove all fat from meat; cut the meat into cubes. Put in food processor; grind to desired consistency.

2. Add remaining ingredients; mix until well blended.

3. Tradition calls for aging this sausage in an airtight container in the refrigerator for 4 days before cooking.

4. Leftover sausage can be stored in the freezer up to 3 months

Nutritional Analysis (per serving, without salt):

Calories: 137 Protein: 15g Carbohydrates: 1g Fat: 8g Saturated Fat: 3g

Cholesterol: 45mg Sodium: 27mg Fiber: 0g

33. Pork Chops with Mustard Cream Sauce

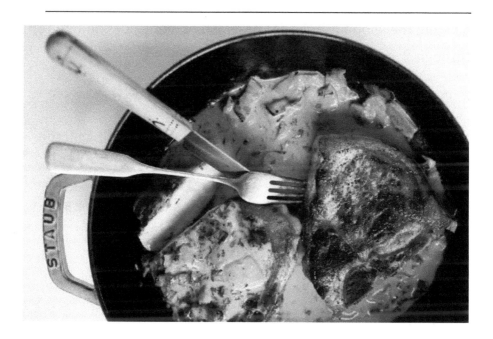

Yields: 4 serving

Ingredients:

- 1 pork chop, 1 inch thick
- 1 tablespoon olive oil
- 1 tablespoon dry white wine
- 1 tablespoon heavy cream
- 1 tablespoon spicy brown mustard or Dijon mustard
- Salt and Pepper

Directions:

1. Salt and pepper the chop on both sides.

2. Heat the oil in a heavy skillet over medium heat.

3. Saute the chop until they're browned on both sides and done through

4. Put the chop on a serving platter, and keep it warm.

5. Put the wine in the skillet, and stir it around, scraping all the tasty brown bits off the pan as you stir.

6. Stir in the cream and mustard, blend well, and cook for a minute or two. Pour over the chop and serve.

34.   Beef and Lentil Chili

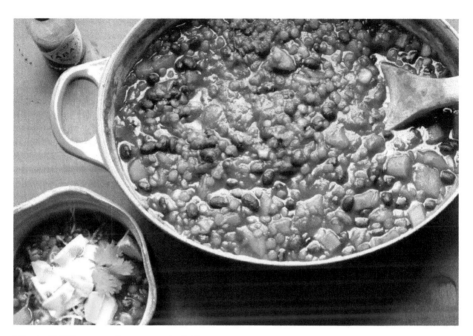

Total Time: 1hr 10 min| Serves 4

Ingredients

- Ground beef – 2 pounds
- Chopped onion – 1
- Chopped stewed potatoes – 2 cans
- Minced cloves garlic – 1
- Chili powder – 3 tablespoons
- Dried and rinsed lentils – 1 cup
- Chili powder – 3 tablespoons

- Chocolate semisweet – 1 ounce
- Tomato sauce – 1 can
- Salt – ¼ teaspoon
- Water – 2 cups

Instructions

1. Use a Dutch oven to cook ground beef and onion over medium heat for 8 minutes or until the meat is pink.

2. Add garlic and then cook for a minute. After that, add the remaining ingredients apart from water and lentils and then cook and bring to a boil.

3. Add lentils and water. Reduce heat and allow to simmer for one hour as you stir often.

4. Serve with a dollop of sour cream, grated cheese or fresh onions.

Nutrients per one serving:

Calories per serving: 367; Carbohydrates: 29g; Protein: 29g; Fat: 16g; Sugar: 4g; Sodium: 655mg; Fiber: 6g

35. Easy Orange Harissa Lamb Chops

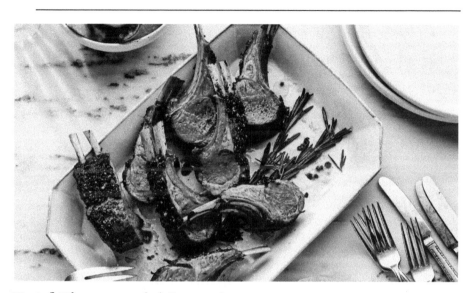

Total Time: 30 min| Serves 6

Ingredients

- Frenched lamb rack – 2.25lm
- Extra virgin olive oil –
- Orange slices for garnish
- Fresh parsley for garnish
- For Spice Mixture
- Harissa spice blend – 2 teaspoons
- Black pepper – 1 teaspoon
- Salt – ½ teaspoon
- Ground coriander -1/2 teaspoon

- Ground cinnamon – ½ teaspoon
- For Marinade
- Zested and juiced orange – 1
- Zested and juiced lemon – 1
- Virgin oil – ¼ cup
- Minced garlic cloves – 10
- Tahini sauce for serving optional

Instructions

1.   In a bowl, combine harissa spice blend, coriander, salt, pepper and cinnamon and then make a spice mixture.

2.   Use the spice mixture to rub on the lamb chops on both sides and then place the lamb chops into a zip lock bag.

3.   Mix the Ingredients for marinade together. Add it into the zip lock bag with the lamb chops. Add the remaining spices into the zip lock as well.

4.   Zip the bag and then use your hands to coat the lamb chops well. Leave it at room temperature for about 20 minutes.

5.   Place a large skillet over medium heat. Add olive oil and heat to shimmering. Add lamb chops to the skillet and then sear for 3 minutes on each side, depending on the thickness of the lamb chops. You can still cook longer as desired.

6.   Transfer the lamb chops to a platter and then cover with foil. Repeat the process with the remaining chops until all are done.

7.   Garnish with fresh parsley leaves and thinly sliced oranges. Add a drizzle of tahini sauce if desired and enjoy.

Nutrients per one serving:

Calories: 132; Carbohydrates: 4g; Protein: 13g; Fat: 8g; Sugar: 2g; Sodium:204mg; Fiber: 1g

36.   Greek Lamb Chops

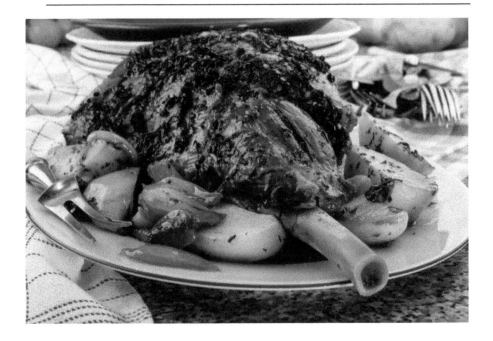

Total Time 18 Mins

Ingredients

- 1/2 teaspoon salt
- 1/2 teaspoon ground cumin
- 1/4 teaspoon ground coriander
- 1/4 teaspoon black pepper
- 1/8 teaspoon ground cinnamon
- 8 (4-ounce) lamb loin chops, trimmed Cooking spray
- 2 tablespoons finely chopped pistachios
- 2 tablespoons chopped fresh flat-leaf parsley
- 1 tablespoon chopped fresh cilantro

- 2 teaspoons grated lemon rind
- 1/8 teaspoon salt 1 garlic clove, minced

Instructions:

1 Heat a large nonstick skillet over medium-high heat. Combine first 5 ingredients; sprinkle evenly over both sides of lamb. Coat pan with cooking spray. Add lamb to pan; cook 4 minutes on each side or until desired degree of doneness.

2 While lamb cooks, combine pistachios and the remaining ingredients; sprinkle over lamb.

Nutrients per one serving:

Calories 233 Fat 11.2g Satfat 3.5g Monofat 5g Polyfat 1.2g Protein 29.6g Carbohydrate 1.9g Fiber 0.8g Cholesterol 90mg Iron 2.4mg Sodium 467mg Calcium 32mg

37.   Beef Tacos

Serves 4

Ingredients*:*

- 2 tablespoons extra virgin olive oil
- 1/2 cup chopped white onion, divided
- 1 cup chopped red bell pepper
- 1 large clove garlic, minced
- 1/2 pound 95%-lean ground beef
- 1/2 teaspoon dried oregano
- 1/4 teaspoon cracked black pepper
- 3/4 cup chopped Roma tomato
- 1 teaspoon chopped jalapeño chile pepper (seeded for less
- heat)
- 4 tablespoons chopped fresh cilantro
- Juice of 1/2 lime
- 8 (6-inch) corn tortillas
- 4 radishes, thinly sliced

Directions:

Heat the oil in a large pan over medium-high heat. Add 1/4
cup of the onion and the bell pepper and garlic, and cook for 30
seconds. Then add the ground beef, breaking up any large

chunks with a spatula. Cook for 5 to 6 minutes, or until the meat is no longer pink. Add the oregano and black pepper while the meat cooks.

In a separate bowl, combine the remaining 1/4 cup chopped onion, tomato, chile pepper, cilantro, and lime juice to make a salsa topping. Mix to incorporate evenly, and set aside.

Warm the tortillas in a flat pan over medium heat. Place two tortillas on four individual plates, scoop the beef mixture onto the tortillas, top with salsa and sliced radishes, fold, and serve.

Nutrition Facts *(amount per serving)*

Calories 294

Total Fat 13 g

Saturated Fat 3 g

Polyunsaturated Fat 2 g

Monounsaturated Fat 5 g

Cholesterol 33 mg

Sodium 73 mg

Potassium 318 mg

Total Carbohydrate 31 g

Dietary Fiber 5 g

Sugars 2 g

Protein 16 g

Calcium 8% • Magnesium 1%

38.   Hearty Beef and Vegetable Soup

8 *Servings*

Ingredients

- 1 tablespoon vegetable oil
- 1 large yellow onion, chopped (2 cups)
- 2 medium carrots, cut into ½-inch dice
- 2 large celery ribs, cut into ½-inch dice
- 2 medium parsnips, cut into ½-inch dice
- 1½ pounds ground sirloin
- 1 quart Homemade Beef Stock (here) or canned low-sodium beef broth 2 cups water
- 1 (14.5-ounce) can no-salt-added canned diced tomatoes in juice, undrained 2
- tablespoons chopped fresh parsley
- 1 teaspoon kosher salt
- ½ teaspoon freshly ground black pepper
- ½ teaspoon dried thyme
- 1 bay leaf
- 2 cups cooked macaroni (optional)

Directions

Heat the oil in a large pot over medium heat. Add the onion, carrots, celery, and parsnips and cook, stirring occasionally, until the onion is softened, about 5 minutes. Push the vegetables to one side of the pot. Put the beef in the empty side of the pot and cook, occasionally stirring and breaking up the meat with the side of a spoon, until the beef loses its raw look, about 5 minutes. Mix the beef and vegetables.

Stir in the broth, water, tomatoes with their juice, parsley, salt, pepper, thyme, and bay leaf. Bring to a boil over high heat. Reduce the heat to medium-low and and bay leaf. Bring to a boil over high heat. Reduce the heat to medium-low and simmer until the vegetables are tender, about 20 minutes. Discard the bay leaf. Ladle into bowls and serve hot.

NUTRITIONAL ANALYSIS

217 calories, 22 g protein, 17 g carbohydrates, 7 g fat, 4 g fiber, 53 mg cholesterol, 395 mg sodium, 712 mg potassium. Food groups: 3 ounces meat, 3 vegetables.

39. Beef and Broccoli

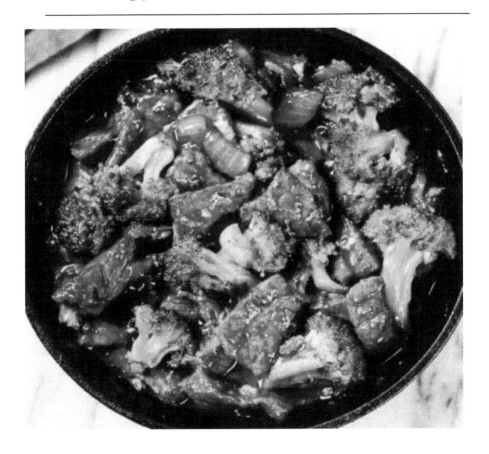

Prep Time: 15 minutes

Cooking Time: 30 minutes

Makes: 7 cups

Ingredients

- 3/4 pound lean ground beef
- 1/4 teaspoon ground ginger

- 3/4 teaspoon garlic powder
- 2 Tablespoons brown sugar
- 1/4 cup low-sodium soy sauce
- 2 teaspoons cornstarch
- 1 Tablespoon sesame oil
- 1/4 teaspoon red pepper flakes
- 1/2 cup water
- 4 cups broccoli, chopped (fresh or frozen)
- 3 cups cooked bulgur

Directions

1. Sauté beef, ginger, and garlic powder in a skillet over medium-high heat until meat is browned.
2. In a bowl, mix sugar, soy sauce, cornstarch, sesame oil, pepper flakes, and water.
3. Add sauce to beef and cook for 5 minutes. Add broccoli and cook until tender.
4. Serve over cooked bulgur.
5. Refrigerate leftovers within 2 hours.

Nutritional Facts

- Calories 364
- Calories from Fat 234
- Fat 26g

- Saturated Fat 16g
- Cholesterol 74mg
- Sodium 559mg
- Potassium 529mg
- Carbohydrates 7g
- Fiber 1g
- Sugar 1g
- Protein 23g
- Vitamin A 355IU
- Vitamin C 51.1mg
- Calcium 36mg
- Iron 3.1mg17

Percent Daily Values are based on a 2000 calorie diet.

40.   Tasty Hamburger Skillet

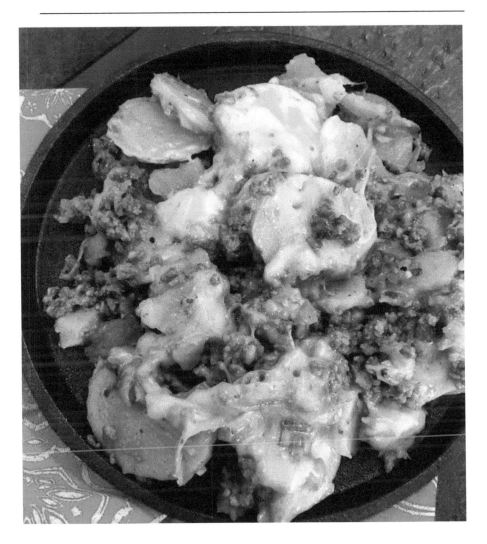

Prep Time: 10 minutes

Cooking Time: 30 minutes

Makes: 9 cups

Ingredients

- 1 pound lean ground beef (15% fat)
- ⅓ cup chopped onion (1/3 medium onion)
- ⅓ cup green pepper, chopped
- 2 cups water
- 1 cup long grain white rice
- 1 teaspoon garlic powder or 4 cloves of garlic
- 1 tablespoon chili powder
- ¼ teaspoon salt
- ¼ teaspoon ground pepper
- 1 can (15 ounces) diced tomatoes, with juice
- 1 ½ cups corn (canned and drained, frozen, or fresh cooked)
- 1 can (15 ounces) red kidney beans, drained and rinsed
- ½ cup grated cheddar cheese

Instructions

1. Cook ground beef, onion, and green pepper in large skillet over medium heat (300 degrees in an electric skillet) until hamburger is no longer pink. Drain excess fat from pan.
2. Add water, rice, garlic powder, chili powder, salt, pepper, tomatoes with juice, corn, and beans.

3. Cook, covered, for about 20 minutes or until rice is soft.

4. Remove from stove top, sprinkle with grated cheese, and serve hot.

5. Refrigerate leftovers within 2 hours.

Notes

1. Garnish this dish with a tablespoon of low-fat sour cream.

2. Flavor boosters: green chilis, jalepeños, more garlic, and other seasonings.

3. Make extra! Leftovers make a great filling for tacos, burritos, filling for stuffed bell peppers, or as a topping for baked potatoes.

4. Use whole grains! Use brown rice instead of white rice and increase cooking time to 45 minutes or until rice is cooked.

5. Cook your own dry beans. One can (15 ounces) is about 1 1/2 to 1 3/4 cups drained beans.

Nutritional Facts

- Calories: 270
- Calories From Fat: 70
- Total Fat: 8g
- Sodium: 240mg

- Carbohydrates: 33g
- Sugars: 3g
- Protein: 16g
- Dietary Fiber: 6g

Percent Daily Values are based on a 2,000 calorie diet. Your daily values may be higher or lower depending on your calorie needs.